I0704639

# Insomnia

## A guide to experiencing a  healthy sleep

**Crown Loveth**

All rights reserved. No part of this publication may be reproduced, distributed, or transmitted in any form or by any means, including photocopying, recording, or other electronic or mechanical methods, without the prior written permission of the publisher, except in the case of brief quotations embodied in critical reviews and certain other noncommercial uses permitted by copyright law.

Copyright © Crown Loveth, 2022

# Table of contents

# Chapter 1

## **What is Insomnia?**

People who struggle to fall asleep are said to have insomnia, sometimes referred to as sleeplessness. If you have insomnia, you may find it difficult to go to sleep, stay asleep, or have a restful night's sleep.

Insomnia is described as "chronic problems with sleep start, duration, consolidation, or quality" in the American Academy of Sleep Medicine's ICSD-3 handbook and when conscious, it has detrimental effects. According to some published polls, between 19% and 50% of individuals report experiencing symptoms of sleeplessness. Insomnia can be short-term, lasting a few days or weeks, or long-term (chronic), lasting more than a month. People who are depressed, anxious, have respiratory problems when they sleep, abuse drugs, and have ongoing health issues are more likely to experience insomnia. The "common cold" of sleep issues is described as insomnia.

Only 21% of women and 25% of men claim to have never had insomnia in their lives. The diagnosis of insomnia is based on two key elements: sleep difficulties that persist despite having enough opportunities for normal sleep and daytime impairment that is a direct result of inadequate sleep quality or duration. Insomnia has a wide range of potential contributing factors and symptoms. It exhausts you and makes it challenging to perform adequately during the day. Anyone can have insomnia, and it can be either the root cause or a symptom of various medical issues.

## Types of Insomnia

### 1. Short-term (Acute) Insomnia

Short-term insomnia is known to frequently be brought on by a recent experience of stress (physical, psychological, or interpersonal), such as an injury, jet lag, life events, or schedule changes. It is known to continue for a few days to a few weeks. The majority of the time, short-term insomnia goes away once the stress has subsided or improved, but it is possible for it to become persistent. Up to 50% of individuals will have occasional short-term insomnia at some time in their life.

### 2. Long term (Chronic) Insomnia

Chronic insomnia is defined as having trouble falling asleep, remaining asleep, or waking up early in the morning and not being able to go back asleep for at least three nights per week for at least three months. Certain actions frequently make chronic sleeplessness worse. For instance, staying in bed too long in an attempt to sleep more soundly may result in nighttime waking and less restorative sleep.

Additionally, this may cause annoyance, worry, and discomfort, all of which have a detrimental effect on one's ability to sleep. The use of alcohol, which impairs the quality of sleep, and daytime naps, which lessen the demand for nighttime sleep, both make insomnia worse.

If you don't have a recognized cause for your insomnia, it is classified as ***primary insomnia***. ***Secondary insomnia*** arises from a medical issue, a prescription side effect, or a chemical like coffee that is disrupting your sleep.

The most common ways that insomnia presents itself are as follows:

- Having trouble falling asleep is referred to as ***sleep-onset insomnia***. This kind of insomnia can affect persons who find it difficult to unwind in bed as well as those whose circadian rhythms are out of whack as a result of things like jet lag or unpredictable job schedules. They awaken sooner than intended; in people with early waking insomnia, sleep onset is generally quick and sleep continuity is good, but awakening is earlier than expected, resulting in insufficient sleep.

- Insomnia that persists after falling asleep is known as ***sleep maintenance insomnia***. This kind of insomnia is prevalent in older sleepers, those who use cigarettes, drink alcohol, or those who take caffeine or alcohol right before bed. Insomnia related to sleep maintenance can also be brought on by conditions like periodic limb movement disorder and sleep apnea. They struggle to fall asleep at first, and this is one of the main features of people with insomnia. In the beginning of the sleep period, they lie in bed yearning to sleep but staying awake for a long time. While some individuals have little trouble falling asleep, they have trouble staying asleep all night. A few moderately extended waking episodes that punctuate the sleep cycle are the hallmark of this type of sleep maintenance insomnia.

- *Mixed insomnia:* Some people experience both problems falling asleep and staying asleep, which is known as mixed insomnia. People who suffer from chronic insomnia may notice that their symptoms change over time.

Both the cognitive and physiological factors contribute to insomnia.

## Cognitive mechanisms

Rumination and hyperarousal may contribute to difficulty falling asleep and may cause a bout of insomnia, according to the cognitive process. When awake, they frequently exhibit restlessness, excessive activity, jitters, and anxiety. That these folks also have trouble sleeping should not come as a surprise. Their arousal-causing physiological processes in the brain and body are stronger and more enduring. They get over-aroused as a result, which increases their level of alertness both during the day and at night. When it's time to go to bed, many people have increased arousal hormone levels and body temperatures.

## Physiological mechanisms

Three key observations in insomniacs serve as the foundation for the physiological mechanism.

The Hypothalamic-Pituitary-Adrenal axis and arousal have been discovered to be active more frequently and catecholamines and cortisol have been found to be elevated in the urine. In addition, patients with insomnia have higher rates of full-body metabolism and heart rate as well as higher global cerebral glucose usage during both awake and NREM sleep. Insomnia may be caused by a dysregulation of the hypothalamic-pituitary-adrenal (HPA) axis, the arousal system, and the cognitive system, according to all of these studies considered together.

# Chapter 2

## Causes of insomnia

Several physical and psychological causes, as well as others, might contribute to insomnia.

- A transient issue, like intermittent stress, is frequently the root reason.
- In other cases, an underlying illness can cause sleeplessness.
- The effects of jet lag, changing shifts at work, or adjusting to any other adjustments to the body's internal clock are common reasons.
- Having an unpleasant bed, a room that was too hot, chilly, or loud, etc.

- Taking recreational drugs, not getting enough exercise, experiencing nightmares or night terrors

Sleep problems are frequently brought on by the signs of another health condition or a seasonal change. For instance, hormonal changes associated with menopause may cause night sweats that may keep you awake.

Changes in the brain cause sleep patterns to be disturbed or altered in patients with Alzheimer's disease.

Fatal familial insomnia is a rare hereditary condition that causes people to have trouble sleeping and can even be fatal in some cases.

# Risk Factors for Insomnia

**1. Age**: Growing older increases your likelihood of experiencing insomnia. Risk factors for insomnia are worse as you get older. Either a medical condition, such as having diabetes, or aging-related changes in the body's intrinsic biological clock (circadian rhythm), are to blame for this.

**2. Genetics and family history**: Some genes may have an impact on sleeping habits and may run in families.

**3. Environment**: The sleep-wake cycle can be impacted by shift work, night work, jet lag, nocturnal light or noise, and uncomfortable high or low temperatures.

**4. Stress**: The risk of sleeplessness is increased by stress. Making it worse is worrying that you won't get enough sleep.

**5. Gender**: Female insomnia is more common than male insomnia, presumably because of hormonal shifts. Additional factors include menopause and pregnancy.

**6. Diseases**: such as Parkinson's disease, Parkinson's-like illness, Parkinson's asthma, chronic pain, sleep apnea, and rheumatoid arthritis

**7. Mental illnesses**: such bipolar disorder, schizophrenia, anxiety disorders, and schizophrenia, among others.

**8. Dietary practices**: such as eating large meals close to bedtime, or abusing coffee or alcohol.

**9. Sleep habit**: Having a sporadic or irregular sleep pattern is one example of an unhealthy sleep routine.

There are a number of unhealthy lifestyle choices that might also raise the risk of insomnia, such as:

- Your sleep schedule is frequently altered.
- Having a sleep interruption.
- Taking protracted naps throughout the day.
- Not enough physical activity
- Using certain drugs, alcohol, nicotine, caffeine, or these substances.

- Using technological gadgets too close to bedtime,

## Insomnia Symptoms

In addition to interrupted sleep, insomnia can cause additional problems, such as:

- Daytime drowsiness or exhaustion
- Irritation, sadness, or anxiousness
- Digestive system issues
- Little energy or motivation
- A lack of focus and attention
- Weak memory
- Hyperactivity and aggressiveness
- Coordination issues that cause mistakes or accidents
- Concern or worry related to sleeping
- Social, professional, or academic difficulty

# Chapter 3

## Complications of Insomnia

Chronic conditions including obesity, diabetes, heart disease, anxiety and depression, asthma, and high blood pressure may be influenced by insomnia.

## Diagnosis of Insomnia

The Athens insomnia scale is frequently used in medicine to assess insomnia. Eight distinct sleep-related characteristics are used to quantify it, and the results are given as a final scale that evaluates a person's entire sleep pattern.

A sleep study or actigraphy can also be used to make the diagnosis.

You can get your insomnia issues diagnosed by a sleep expert. The following can be asked:

- Inquiry about your health history, sleeping habits, and consumption of alcohol and illicit substances.

- They can also look for underlying issues with a test

- A sleep test can be done overnight to track your sleeping habits.

- Put on a tracker that monitors motion and sleep-wake cycles.

- Depending on your sleep-wake cycle and amount of daytime drowsiness, a questionnaire may be required of you. Keeping a sleep journal for a few weeks can also be required of you.

# Chapter 4

**Insomnia and stress**

Stress and insomnia are two conditions that have a close relationship and seem to be connected on a pathophysiological level. Stress raises the risk of insomnia, insomnia exacerbates stress, and the presence of both elements has a detrimental effect on the prognosis of each condition. A number of predisposing personality traits operate as a mediator between stressful life events and the development of chronic insomnia.

Stressful life events frequently cause insomnia problems, and hyperarousal caused by physiological and cognitive-emotional processes can disrupt sleep and cause chronic insomnia.

Situational insomnia can result from a lack of sleep in reaction to a particular stressful environment. It has been demonstrated that extreme sleep interruptions in reaction to stress may be a sign of sensitivity to insomnia even in the absence of a history of sleep disorders.

## How does stress cause insomnia and affect our sleep ?

A healthy life cycle for all the processes occurring inside of us is only guaranteed by the biological clock that exists in our body. This chain is broken by stress, which has a detrimental effect on your quality of life in many different ways. The stress level system is taken over by the brain when you are feeling anxious and exhausted, filling your body with hormones that make you want to fight and freeze. The pulse and blood pressure rise when cortisol and adrenocorticotropic hormones flow through the vines. Then, all of a sudden, your body becomes hyper aroused and goes into alert. Your body is vulnerable to even the slightest noises and discomforts in this condition.

## How to know your insomnia is stress induced ?

Insomnia brought on by stress is when you can't fall asleep because of your stress and worry levels. It may be a clue that your insomnia is related to your stress levels if you experience sleeping issues while you are experiencing periods of intense stress and worry. A doctor may be consulted in order to receive a formal diagnosis of insomnia, and he or she will likely ask you several questions and/or have you keep a sleep diary. Your thoughts may be busy at night from worries. Your anxiety may be exacerbated by problems at work, school, or with your family. Your ability to sleep may be affected by this. Stress and worry can continue for a long time after traumatic events like a loved one's death, a divorce, or a job loss. A prolonged lack of sleep may result from this conditions.

## Managing stress induced insomnia

Anxiety and stress are strong disruptors of sleep. Avoid such activities before they start interfering with your sleep if the things you do before night (or while you're in bed) make you feel nervous, whether it's watching the news, sending work emails, or browsing through your social media feeds.

A shift in perspective could help you unwind and sleep better if stress is keeping you up at night. This strategy has the advantage of being able to help break the link between stress and sleeplessness. You may be able to see chances you may have overlooked by approaching a topic from many perspectives.

It is possible to alter your viewpoint on a stressful circumstance by engaging in cognitive restructuring, which entails understanding and altering your thinking patterns.

Numerous health and stress-reduction advantages come from journaling too.

In the cycle of stress and insomnia, writing may help you declutter your thoughts, work through the emotions that are keeping you up at night, and come up with ideas and create strategies to help you deal with the stressful events.

Decide to use your bedroom largely for sleeping so that you link it with calm and rest rather than tension.

These routines or behaviors can assist you in maintaining a regular sleep schedule in addition to avoiding anxiety triggers:

- Even on weekends, get up and fall asleep at the same hour every day.

- Walk and other low-impact exercises are good forms of regular exercise (but avoid vigorous exercise too close to bedtime, which tends to wake up and energize your body)

- Do not take extended or repeated naps.

- Cut back on your alcohol and caffeine consumption.

- Avoid large meals before going to bed.

- Making a regular nighttime routine can also be beneficial since it sends a message to your body and mind that it is time to go to sleep. Yours may involve performing some mild yoga while listening to music, or it can involve having a shower followed by reading a book.

# Chapter 5

## Insomnia and children

However, from a clinical perspective, the most common manifestations of childhood insomnia, particularly in younger children, are bedtime refusal or struggles, difficulty falling asleep after "lights out," or frequent or prolonged night wakings requiring parental intervention. In general, the working definition of insomnia in children may be construed as similar to that in adults, significant difficulty initiating or maintaining sleep.

The most prevalent behavioral sleep condition affecting young children is behavioral insomnia of childhood (BIC), which is characterized by issues with bedtime and nocturnal wakings. Children who have insomnia exhibit noncompliant nighttime behaviors such as vocal protestations, unwillingness to go to sleep, and recurrent demands and, they get up during the night frequently and for a lengthy time, necessitating caregiver assistance to get them back to sleep.

## Causes of insomnia in children

Insomnia in children can have many different root causes, including behavioral problems as well as medical conditions, and is frequently brought on by a combination of these factors. The negative effects of medications, such as antidepressants and those used to treat attention deficit hyperactivity disorder (ADHD), can also make kids have insomnia. Other health problems, it can be a sleep issue, such as sleep apnea or restless legs syndrome, or it might be brought on by symptoms of allergies, growing pains, or dermatitis, such as itchy skin.

## Risk Factors for Insomnia in children

The amount of sweet food consumed during the day or watching TV immediately before bed, for instance, might be enough to prevent your child from falling asleep.

Young children not only suffer stress, but tension that is frequently brought on by problems at home or at school can lead to insomnia.

Caffeine is a stimulant that can keep youngsters up at night and is included in many sodas and energy beverages. After lunch, try to minimize your child's intake. Better still, make every effort to avoid consuming these drinks altogether.

## Treatment for insomnia in children

Children seldom "outgrow" sleep and bedtime issues when they are mistreated; instead, they can become chronic.

Treatments that focus on behavior, however, can have positive outcomes that last. Behavioral factors are frequently to blame for a child's nighttime reluctance and can be changed through behavioral strategies also.

- Prior to going to bed, set a regimen that is reliable and excludes anything stimulating, like watching TV.

- Introduce the kid to more suitable sleep associations that they can access easily at night, such as the usage of a transitional toy (eg, blanket, stuffed animal).

- Encourage your young child to learn self-soothing techniques so they can go to sleep at night without their parents' help.

- Use the technique of "bedtime fading," which includes temporarily setting the child's bedtime at the time at which they typically fall asleep and then gradually moving that time forward.

- Reduce the amount of time spent correcting children for bad bedtime habits like delaying and extra demands.

- Offer rewards, such as stickers for staying in bed, as positive reinforcement for acceptable conduct.

- Teach older kids cognitive-behavioral approaches for relaxing on their own, which can also be helpful.

# Chapter 6

## Treatment and Management of Insomnia

By practicing good sleep hygiene, insomnia can be controlled. Cognitive behavioral therapy for insomnia (CBT-I), a 6- to 8-week treatment program that teaches you how to fall asleep more quickly and stay asleep longer, is typically suggested as the first line of treatment for chronic insomnia and can be very successful when carried out properly. Additionally, effective drugs such benzodiazepines, agonists of benzodiazepine receptors, melatonin receptor agonists, and antagonists of the orexin receptor are utilized as therapies.

Insomnia can have a variety of causes, and the best course of action will depend on these factors.

## A. Sleep hygiene

A set of rules known as "sleep hygiene" encourages restful sleep and includes the following:

1. Pick a certain wake-up time. Regardless of how much sleep you get the night before, wake up at the same time every day.

2. Pick a time for going to bed. Decide on the earliest bedtime that will allow you to obtain the rest you require. A good bedtime is one that allows you to receive the sleep you need but keeps you from staying in bed for too long. Too much time in bed,

however, will result in lighter, more erratic sleep. Only occupy your bed for as long as you truly need to sleep.

3. Get into bed when you feel tired, but not earlier than your preferred bedtime. Wait till you are drowsy before going to bed. Therefore, if you are still awake at the time you've set for going to bed, give it a little more time till you're ready to sleep.

4. If you can't sleep, get out of bed. If you're having trouble falling asleep while laying in bed, get up and do something calming outside of your bedroom. After calming yourself by reading a book, watching TV, or engaging in another activity, return to bed when you are able to nod off easily. Once more, if you have trouble falling asleep, get

up. This cycle should be repeated until you nod off. When you have trouble falling asleep, both before bed and during the night, you need to get out of bed.

5. Avoid worrying or making plans while you are asleep. Don't stress or make plans for the next day when you're laying in bed at night. Set aside a different period of the day to complete these tasks. When you go into bed, if you instantly start thinking and fretting, get out of bed and wait until your thoughts aren't interfering with falling asleep before returning. You can break the habit of thinking in bed.

6. You should only use your bed to sleep. Rest in your bed at all times. In other words, refrain from engaging in other activities like

eating, watching television, or doing your schoolwork.

7. Take no naps. No naps, as they will prevent you from falling asleep when it is time for bed.

## B. Home care techniques

Many treatments and advice can support managing insomnia. They entail adjustments to:

### Sleeping patterns

- Set a schedule by going to bed and waking up at the same time.
- Before going to bed, avoid using any screen-equipped devices.

- Start unwinding, for instance, by taking a bath one hour before going to bed.
- Keep phones and other electronics away from your bed.
- Before going to bed, make sure the room is at a comfortable temperature. To make a space darker, use drapes or blackout shades.

**Dietary practices**

- Avoid eating before bed. If you need to, have a nutritious snack before going to bed.
- But stay away from having a substantial meal two to three hours before bed.
- Reduce your intake of alcohol and caffeine, especially at night.

- Eat a balanced, healthy diet to improve your overall well being.

**Addressing other health concerns**

One or more more pillows might be used to elevate the upper body for anyone suffering from acid reflux or a cough.

## C. Calming exercises

- Regular exercise is advised, but avoid it four hours before bed.
- Practice deep breathing and relaxation techniques, especially before bed.
- Find a calming activity to do before bed, like reading or listening to music.

## D. Therapy using cognitive behavior (CBT-i)

Although prescription drugs may be used occasionally to treat persistent insomnia, cognitive behavioral therapy for insomnia (CBTi), a kind of psychotherapy or talk therapy, is widely regarded as the gold standard of care. As a first-line treatment for persistent insomnia, CBT is typically advised.

Through CBTi, your body and brain are effectively being taught new sleeping habits. People who suffer from persistent insomnia grow to dislike their beds, bedrooms, and sleeping itself. Through instruction in strategies that especially target the psychological aspects of insomnia, such as feeling negative emotions and fears about being unable to go asleep, CBTi attempts to eliminate that resistance.

In addition to other complementary therapies that can aid in sleep, CBTi can include breathing exercises, activities for muscular relaxation, and other methods. In order to encourage restful sleep, it may also be necessary to alter your sleep schedule or bedroom setting.

CBT-I, as opposed to sleeping medicines, aids in overcoming the root reasons of your insomnia. When it comes to treating persistent insomnia, research has shown that CBT is as effective as or perhaps better than sleep aids.

The following are a few of the CBT-I, or CBT-I techniques, that are explicitly targeted towards treating insomnia:

**Psychological methods**

Before going to bed, writing down worries or concerns in a diary might prevent someone from actively trying to solve them while still trying to sleep. It is necessary to alter the negative attitudes and beliefs that an insomniac has formed about sleep as a result of previous unfavorable experiences if they are to change their sleep patterns.

Thinking things like, "This is dreadful, and I fear going to bed since I won't be able to sleep. Many insomniacs utter phrases like "I can't sleep and I'll be a mess tomorrow!

Changing these negative beliefs to more positive ones needs cognitive restructuring. Examples of such positive thinking are "Even if it takes a little time to fall asleep, I'll be OK tomorrow" and "I can let go and believe in my body's natural capacity to sleep."

## Stimulus management

This requires changing the habits that train your mind to resist sleep. The chronic insomniacs develop an association between their bed and bedroom and worry and alertness as a result of repeated episodes of difficulty falling asleep in bed. The insomniac is instructed by CBT-i to just use their bed for sleeping and having sex in order to break this conditioned link. Reading, watching TV, talking on the phone, eating, drinking, using the computer, and other activities should all be done in a different room. Setting up a wake-up and sleep schedule is another component of this approach.

The insomniac is advised to move to another room and participate in a soothing activity until he/she falls asleep if, after turning out the light, he/she is unable to fall asleep in 10 minutes. Then should return to his/her bed and fall asleep once he/she is tired.

**Sleep limitation**
Many people with insomnia struggle to fall asleep for hours in bed. They thus worry about their ability to go asleep, stay asleep, and, in the event that they awaken, return to sleep. By going to bed sooner and remaining

in bed longer in an effort to obtain more sleep, they frequently make issues worse. As a result, they wind up staying up in bed later trying to fall asleep.

Your time in bed is restricted as part of this therapy, and naps are also forbidden. It is intended to deprive you of adequate sleep so that you are exhausted when it is time for bed and can doze off quickly and soundly. As you get better at sleeping, you eventually spend more time in bed.

**Relaxation methods**

The insomniac can let go and drift off to sleep using methods that calm the mind and relax the body. Slow, deep breathing and increasing relaxation assist calm the nervous system and produce sleeping-friendly environments. Patients can learn to notice their thoughts objectively by engaging in mindfulness exercises, such as mindfulness meditation. For lowering emotional reactivity, clearing the mind, and preparing for sleep, this technique is quite beneficial.

You may relax by releasing your muscles, managing your breathing and pulse rate, and using other techniques like yoga, meditation, and breathing exercises.

## Contradictory motive

In contrast to anticipating going to sleep, this tactic emphasizes staying awake while in bed. It facilitates a decrease in tension and stress about difficulty sleeping. Learned insomnia is the condition for which it works best.

## Constrained arousal

Recognizing and getting rid of behaviors that you may have formed to help you sleep better but are no longer helpful. Thus lowering causes of increased arousal, such as sleep-related anxiety.

# Chapter 7

## Conclusion

This book covers many aspects that needed to be known about insomnia to give you enough knowledge and leverage to correctly diagnose and treat the condition with ease and put an end to its hold over you, or your children or a family member.

After reading the book, the best way to make the knowledge you acquired useful is to practice it. So make sure to put each strategy to successfully manage and treat insomnia in action and enjoy results.

**Now say hello to an insomnia free life....**

www.ingramcontent.com/pod-product-compliance
Lightning Source LLC
Chambersburg PA
CBHW071552260726
48653CB00007BA/2961